FITNESS
VEGETARIAN
DIET

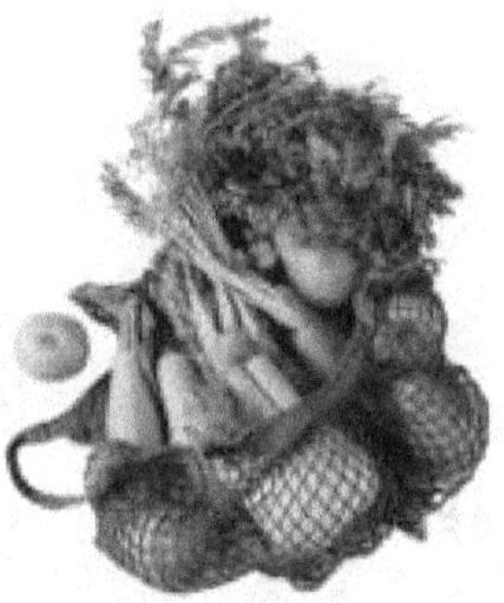

Eating Right for a Healthy and Active Lifestyle as a Vegan.

Cathryn D. Dutton

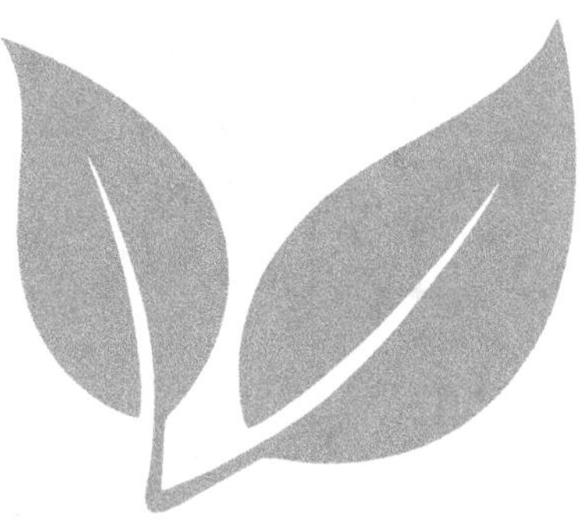

Table Of Content

INTRODUCTION

Once upon a time, there was a woman named Lucy who decided that she wanted to lead a healthier lifestyle. She started researching different ways to improve her overall health and came across the idea of becoming a vegetarian. She was intrigued by the idea as it could provide her with an abundance of health benefits.

Lucy started to make the transition to a vegetarian lifestyle and decided to incorporate fitness into her routine as well. She started to go for walks, runs and even joined a yoga studio. She was amazed at how much her body was responding to the new changes. She was feeling more energized and was losing weight as well.

Lucy continued to refine her new lifestyle, ensuring that she was eating a balanced vegetarian diet and getting enough exercise. She soon discovered that she felt better than she had ever felt before. She was able to stay active and healthy while still enjoying her favorite vegetarian dishes.

Lucy was so happy with her newfound energy and health that she decided to spread the word about her journey. She started writing blogs and articles about her experience and soon had many people following her journey.

Lucy's transformation has been truly inspiring and she has been able to show people that it is possible to be a fitness vegetarian and still lead a healthy lifestyle. She hopes to continue to inspire others and help them realize that they too can make healthy changes in their lives.

Accepting and making changes are never simple, and switching to a vegetarian diet is more difficult than you might think.

So, it is crucial to do a thorough examination before adjusting to a new lifestyle Occasionally switching to a vegetarian diet might be difficult. Consequently, it is preferable to be aware of both the positive and bad effects in advance.

because giving up meat is only one aspect of becoming a vegetarian.

There are many different types of vegetarians; some enjoy eating fish, while others do not. On the other hand, there are people who only eat fruits and vegetables and even avoid dairy items like cheese and eggs.

A vegetarian diet is always a matter of personal preference.

When avoiding cottage cheese and other nutritious meals that offer vital nutrients, one must also consider the nutritional supplements that the body would need.

It is advisable to begin gradually and transition to a strict vegetarian diet over time. Although it may be hard to imagine, there will be significant changes throughout the entire system because the body won't be receiving something it is very accustomed to.
It is always preferable to lower the amount gradually rather than abruptly eliminating meat from the diet. Instead, substitute fish or chicken for the meat and start fresh.
gradually reducing consumption, eventually becoming a vegetarian.

Understanding the nutritional content of the foods that will be eaten in place of meat is the most important part of deciding to live a vegetarian lifestyle.

Those who disagree with a vegetarian lifestyle typically think that if meat were excluded from the diet, their bodies would be deficient in important vitamins and minerals. Yet, many people have been successful in making the transition to a vegetarian diet. By giving their bodies the nutrients they needed, these people have been able to make up for the gap left by a vegetarian diet.

 Many studies have demonstrated that green vegetables like broccoli, kale, and spinach contain astronomical quantities of calcium and that eating these veggies regularly will provide the nutrients needed to maintain good health.
Nuts are also widely known for being a good source of protein. Such vegetarian diets might make sure that a person receives enough to live a healthy life with a balanced diet.

Making the switch to a vegetarian diet is among the most crucial things you can do to ensure that your body feels healthy. And those who already follow a vegan diet must have noticed how wonderful they feel, how much energy they have, and how simple it is to shed pounds.without depriving themselves. So begin to consider this and go closer to a fulfilling live.

CHAPTER 1:

Getting Started as a Vegetarian

It may seem ridiculous to think about the steps one would need to take to figure out how to adopt a vegetarian diet.

Yet it's not as easy as just cutting off meat from one's diet, is it? That simple question has a simple answer: not really. Some believe that becoming a vegan involves considerably more work than merely abstaining from meat products like steak or hamburgers.

In order to stay fit and avoid depriving one's body of something that it fundamentally needs to function completely in the way it was intended to, one would learn that examining the idea of becoming a vegan demands a lot of research and significant effort.

. When switching to a vegan diet, the most crucial thing to remember to do is to go slowly. A relaxed approach won't make much of a difference if you've been accustomed to eating meat for years.
To become a vegan, you will need to put in some serious and thought-out effort. Start by progressively reducing the amount of meat in your daily diet.

You can go without meat for a few days before replacing it with fish or chicken. When the body gradually adjusts to the change in diet, this procedure can eventually assist you in giving up meat permanently.

In order to ensure that their body is getting the nutrients it needs to be well-built and efficient, a person who wants to learn how to adopt a lacta-vegetarian diet will also need to conduct a small amount of research into the nutrients that are included in various vegetables. It is important to remember that nutrients such as B and C vitamins, iron, and zinc are necessary for human health.

A proportional diet must also include foods high in calcium and protein, thus it is important to understand the nutritional content of the food you are eating. Making ensuring the body receives all the vital nutrients and vitamins it needs to function properly is important.

People must make sure they get enough protein into their bodies because they are cutting meat out of their diets. Protein is essential for the human body, thus those learning how to become vegans will want to find alternative sources of protein so that their bodies can function as they were meant to.

Healthy Vegetarian Eating

Vegan diets are recognized to be incredibly wholesome and hearty, yet when someone follows a normal diet and is a vegetarian, it typically doesn't draw much attention. When someone cuts out animal protein and red meat from their diet, they are cutting out a major source of protein that their body needs. It follows that a vegan's diet must include items that are nutrient-dense and typically found in meat products if they are to be healthy.By exploring a diet consisting of fruits, vegetables, and whole grains, people can easily avail the vitamins and nutrients they want from vegetarian sources so that their vegetarian way of life is healthy and in proportion.

One can get the necessary protein content they need for growth by eating foods like eggs, almonds, soy products, and legumes. It's also important to remember that vegans require a similar amount of other nutrients, including the vitamins D and B12, the minerals calcium and iron, and the vitamin D.

Yet, it is true that cutting out meat and replacing it with a diet high in vegetables, fruits, and whole grains is healthful. But, vegetarians must also worry about other important elements, such as getting the correct ratio of vitamins and minerals in their diet.

While many people regularly take vitamin supplements, many devout vegetarians avoid doing so because many of these supplements contain animal products. A healthy lacto-vegetarian diet must include foods high in vitamins B and C, iron, and niacin because these nutrients are also essential to this way of life.

While choosing to become a vegan, one need not sacrifice their health. Consuming a nutritious vegetarian diet is not simple. One must set aside time only for leisurely research to identify foods that contain the nutrients the body needs the most. You might need to read a lot of books, magazines, or even the internet to learn about this.

When someone isn't eating anymore, they can replace meat in their diet with a variety of other foods. For instance, one can opt for soy milk as an alternative to cow's milk which in turn will provide the necessary calcium to the body. Including nuts and grains into a vegetarian diet suitably turns it into a healthy diet Moreover, grains and nuts are rich in proteins that support the growth of strong bones.

 When people stop eating, they can replace meat in their diets with a variety of other foods. For instance, one can choose soy milk instead of cow's milk, which would help the body get the necessary calcium. A vegetarian diet can be made nutritious by adding nuts and grains to it. Moreover, grains and nuts are rich in proteins that support the growth of strong bones.

Several studies have shown that vegetarians typically follow a balanced eating plan that results in a physically fit and healthy physique. Also, they are more likely to stay active and healthy. People must pay close attention to the nutrients included in the foods they eat and make sure to eat a balanced diet if they want to maintain a healthy vegan diet.

CHAPTER 2:

vegetarian diet for losing weight

Because they need to lose weight yet detest the thought of starving themselves, many people decide to become vegetarians.

Because you are eliminating all red meat from your diet, which can include a lot of fat that is stored in your body's cells and contributes to weight gain, going vegetarian can help you lose weight in a variety of other ways as well. A vegetarian consumes a lot of healthful foods like fruits, vegetables, fish, and shellfish, all of which can help you lose weight. You should really think about switching to a vegetarian lifestyle because dieting is challenging when you want to lose weight. Since vegetables are healthy and naturally low in calories, you won't have to worry about gaining weight while eating them. Fruits are nutritious for you, but because the body likes to retain water, they are also quite high in water content and can cause you to weigh extra.

A solid, well-rounded vegetarian diet designed for maximum weight loss includes a variety of tasty foods and satiating spices. You know, the way we prepare food and the ingredients we use can make it fattening.

Even if you eat a bowlful of nutritious mushrooms, cooking them in butter and heavy cream to make a soup will add calories and nullify their naturally beneficial effects.

As far as possible, avoid frying your food if you're following a vegetarian diet to lose weight. If you want to sauté any of your vegetables, use extra virgin olive oil, or EVOO as Rachel Ray calls it. This oil has fewer calories and some of the healthy fats your body requires.

Moreover, you should avoid high-fat cheeses and choose lower-fat types, as well as look at alternatives like substituting plain yogurt for sour cream.

A vegetarian diet is a healthy way to eat and an excellent tool for losing weight. We're prepared to wager that you'll keep up your vegetarian diet once you reach your weight loss objectives.

Being a vegetarian is easier than many people realize. If you cultivate the majority of your vegetables, you'll notice that you have more energy, a faster metabolism (which burns fat), and lower food costs.

Hence, choose a vegetarian diet for optimum weight reduction and watch the pounds melt off without constantly feeling hungry.

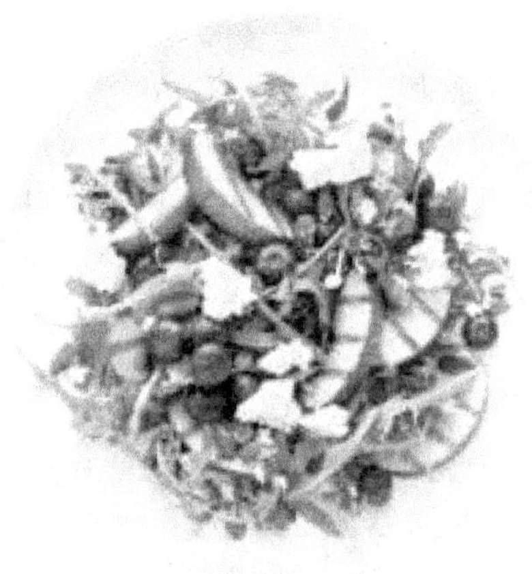

Vegetarain diet lossing weight

CHAPTER 3:

Having a vegetarian diet

Being a vegetarian is really healthy. In addition to aiding in the recovery of internal metabolism, it finally results in a significantly healthier way of life.

We frequently encounter neighbors who need to change their diets because they have a condition that may have been brought on by an unhealthy diet. Being a vegetarian could aid someone in maintaining a careful eye on their health because those who eat meat are more likely to develop diabetes and high cholesterol.

Vegetarians are typically thought to consume a lot of green salad, but this perception is partly mistaken because, from a larger viewpoint, the categorisation is very different from what is typically thought.

The few mentioned classifications are shown below:

• Lacto-ovo-vegetarians – Those who favor eating both dairy and eggs. The vegetarian diet that is most frequently chosen by vegetarians.

• Lacto-vegetarians – Those who fall into this category eat dairy products but no eggs.

• Vegans are those who don't eat any dairy products, eggs, or other animal products.

• Fruitarians are classified as vegans when they consume the fewest processed foods possible while still maintaining an optimal level of nutrition. It primarily consists of uncooked fruits, grains, and nuts. Fruitarians only consume food that can be picked without harming the plant, according to their philosophy.

• Macrobiotic – Those who follow this diet do so for moral and intellectual reasons. With an understanding of the positive and negative energy that food contains, it is taken into account. The yin is its positive quality, whereas the yang is its adverse quality. This eating pattern seeks to keep up a healthy diet. This diet becomes more specialized after ten levels.

Although though vegetarians make up the majority of the population, eliminating all animal products and, in certain extreme circumstances, even fruits and vegetables, results in a diet that solely contains brown rice.

Everyone has different motivations for being a vegetarian. For example, some people do it because they don't want to harm animals, while others do it because they believe it to be a healthier lifestyle choice. Whatever the cause, vegetarians live far healthier lives than non-vegetarians, as demonstrated by medical research.

A vegetarian is less likely to get diabetes, high cholesterol, or even some types of cancer. When food is cultivated organically with little use of pesticides, the risk of ingesting hazardous chemicals—about which scientists have shown to cause significant damage to the proper functioning of the body and neurological system—is eliminated.

If this has in any way persuaded you to follow a vegetarian diet, go ahead and take the first step toward a much better life. Although initially fairly demanding and difficult, it would eventually lead to enormous advances that would make people much safer and healthier.

CHAPTER 4

Sport Nutrition for Vegetarian

Let's imagine that despite being a vegan and being quite active in sports, you are concerned about eating the correct foods.

Not to worry. You may maintain a vegetarian lifestyle and engage in physical activity while getting all the nourishment you require. Just because you don't want to eat meat doesn't mean you have to change your diet.

In fact, you could discover that a vegetarian diet makes it quite easy for you to engage in physical activity because the nutrients in grains, vegetables, and other plant foods really offer you greater energy.

The first thing you should keep in mind is that you must eat before exercising so that your body can start processing the food and provide you with the nutrition you need to survive a rigorous workout and have the energy to engage in the sports you enjoy.

This means that vegetarians must consume a lot of carbs prior to engaging in physical activity so that the nutrients found in those foods can do its job.

In order to replace the nutrition that is naturally lost through sweat during your workout, you should have a healthy vegetarian meal right after you finish engaging in your sport.

But, you should try to limit the amount of carbohydrates you eat at this meal because they can quickly turn into fat, negating all the advantages you have just given yourself.

If you are a lacto-vegetarian who participates in a lot of physical activity, we advise you to consume a lot of nuts, grains, and fruits, all of which are rich in carbs and can help your body.

water that you will eventually sweat out during your athletic session.

Since exercise is so crucial to staying in shape, vegetarian athletes frequently worry about their diet. What they actually need to keep in mind is that certain vitamins and minerals are necessary for the body to operate properly. When it comes to it, research is important.

In order to prevent their nutrition from suffering, ask some of your vegetarian friends what they do prior to participating in sports. Search online for tips on how to maximize the nutrition in your vegetarian diet before engaging in physical activity.

If you're a vegetarian who does a lot of sports and you're concerned about nutrition, read books and see your doctor along the way. You can never have too much information, so look for what's available to you and then pay attention. In the end, it will all be worthwhile!

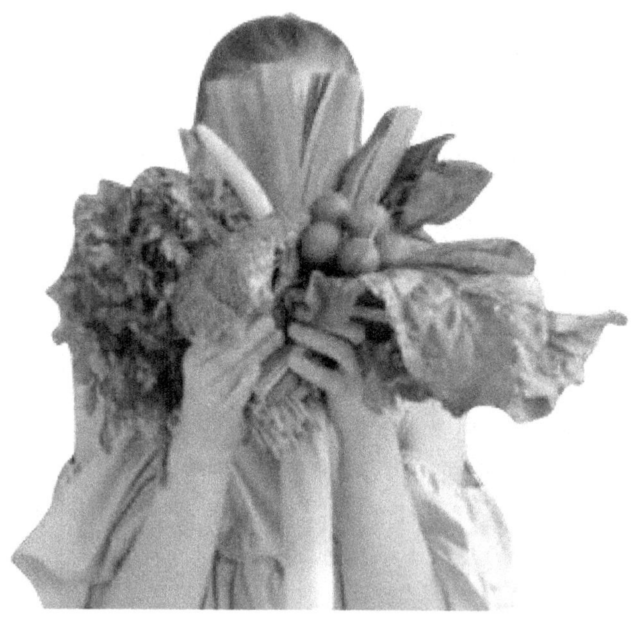

CHAPTER 5:

Cooking Vegetarian for Everyone

It is true that cooking vegetarian meals is among the simplest skills to learn. Vegetarian food is very interesting and simple to prepare, even for those who are afraid of boiling water or cooking food.

Everyone can cook vegetarian food. In addition to being highly nutritious, vegetarian cooking is simple for everyone.

The best-selling book "Vegetarian Cooking for Everyone" was just released by America's top chef, Deborah Madison. You shouldn't consider it to be another cookbook for vegetarians. It includes 800 scrumptious recipes as well as crucial information on the elements and techniques of cooking.

Both well-known dishes like guacamole and lesser-known ones like green lentils with roasted veggies are taught in unique ways in this book.

Both well-known dishes like guacamole and lesser-known ones like green lentils with roasted veggies are taught in unique ways in this book.

Cashew curry, preserved lemons, and beets. The book is freely accessible everywhere and costs only $26.40 on Amazon.com.

The 124-page chapter on veggies, titled "The Heart of Matter," can be used as a reference for any vegetarian culinary abilities, according to an Amazon review. It might have been used as a guide or as assistance when purchasing veggies. Madison offers equally creative recipes and advice for various types of foods, including grains, soy, dairy products, and sweets.

It has proven to be an excellent resource and has made learning enjoyable for all of its readers. One reviewer even admitted that the author's writing about recipes for the typical kitchen is what draws readers of all ages. It's not like those chef books where the reader or student finds it challenging to prepare the recipes.

The book "Vegetarian Cookery for Everyone" is written for all readers. Even a mediocre cook who reads from it can plan or cook good meals. A novice or new learner who can successfully create tasty vegetarian meals will find this to be of great assistance as it will boost his confidence. It has been determined that "Vegetarian Cooking for Everyone" is a thorough book that is interesting to everyone, including those who want to use it as a resource for regular cooking. Every meal is covered, including appetizers, sizzlers, snacks, breakfast, lunch, and supper.

It's easy to find the ingredients in one's cupboard and refrigerator, and using them to make something delicious is quite satisfying and enjoyable.

This book teaches everyone the fundamentals of vegetarian cookery. So read the book and have fun!

Gourmet Vegetarian Cooking

There are a ton of chances for vegans who enjoy preparing upscale foods to explore and discover. You can prepare a large variety of epicurean vegan foods in a variety of settings and circumstances; you simply need to look for opportunities.
Unfortunately, due to space restrictions, we are unable to list every cookbook available in this brief post. Nonetheless, there are a few suggestions I can make for great vegetarian food preparation.

First, let's define an epicurean meal. Now, the issue of feasibility arises. A gourmet lunch is actually a special meal without meat or pasta that involves combining intriguing and uncommon ingredients to create dishes that are not only delicious but also visually stunning.

Gourmet can be defined in a variety of ways, but making gourmet vegan food requires a certain level of skill. It demands a lot of flavor and the capacity to transform ordinary components into works of beauty.

So what information is required to prepare a gourmet vegetarian meal? If they have been a lacto-vegetarian for a while, they may want to think about what they enjoy eating and how to add creativity to make it interesting and delectable in addition to scrumptious.

The greatest method for introducing vegetarian food to individuals is to think about the kinds of gourmet meals they have previously enjoyed. It is absolutely true that practically all of us have eaten vegetarian meals. It's important to always explore for methods to make a dish without the meat and keep the flavor intact.

We know almost everyone can do this with a little creativity and ingenuity!

In their neighborhood bookstore, on various websites, and online, one can find sizable and varied recipe books that are wholly devoted to gourmet vegetarian way of cooking. Search for culinary techniques that use ingredients that all find fascinating before trying the dish.

If they begin from anywhere, many people will not be able to prepare a gourmet vegetarian feast. Yet, if you strictly adhere to the directions, you can avoid a culinary disaster.

As a vegan chef, preparing a gourmet dinner may be a truly adventurous and revitalizing experience. Many people think that living a vegetarian lifestyle requires confusion and curiosity. When one can simply show that they are capable of providing a vegetarian banquet that is exquisite, visually appealing, and delicious, they may just wave them over to their side of the fence.

But don't push yourself too far. A lacto-vegetarian lifestyle is not for everyone. The best thing someone can do is cook from the heart and stick to their commitment to leading a vegetarian lifestyle, which involves creating gourmet dishes that taste like they contain mutton but don't actually contain any meat.

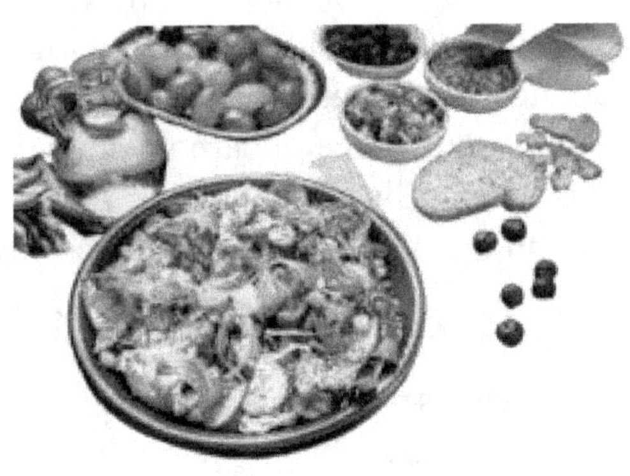

CHAPTER 6

Low Carbohydrate Vegetarian

The body needs a variety of nutrients to stay healthy. Being a vegetarian is beneficial, but you must carefully balance the vitamins and nutrients.

The carbohydrate balance should be the only thought that enters your head.

Only because carbs are such a tremendous source of energy should they be consumed in moderation. An excessive amount of carbohydrates in a vegetarian diet will cause the body to produce fat. Carbs change sugar, which then turns into fat, which might be problematic if there is an excessive amount of conversion.

If you want to reduce your intake of carbohydrates, you should limit your intake of foods high in carbohydrates such rice, potatoes, and cereals. While these foods are a good source of carbohydrates, it is also not suggested to fully exclude them from your diet. The consumption of certain food products needs to be reduced.

Moreover, flour contains carbs, including whole wheat flour. If you are serious about getting the right amount of carbohydrates, you should avoid or limit eating bread. To control the right consumption of carbohydrates, ensure that the source of your carbohydrates is acceptable. Eat whole grain bread instead of white bread to satisfy your body's need for carbohydrates.

Being a vegetarian is beneficial, but it requires a lot of sacrifices. There should be a large amount of fresh, green vegetables in the diet.

Also, consideration should be given to the choice of oils used in food preparation. To get the necessary amount of carbs, you must use the right amount of olive oil. To guarantee a reduced carb intake, also take into account steaming and grilling with oil. Green and leafy veggies contain natural vitamins. Avoid consuming carbs that will cause you to gain weight.

The decision to choose a vegetarian diet varies among individuals for a variety of reasons. The primary motivation is shedding additional weight. Some are really concerned about the slaughter of numerous animals. The main requirement for leading a vegetarian lifestyle is a healthy diet. An excessive intake of carbs can convert to sugar, which can progressively result in weight gain.

You must be very careful to determine the precise amount of carbohydrates available in your diet before beginning a vegetarian diet that is similarly low in carbohydrate content. Low carbohydrate intake may have an impact on your body, and most crucially, your health. Nutrition is the most crucial component of a healthy diet.

Recipes for Low-Calorie Vegetarian Food

Perhaps someone who wanted to lose weight would have preferred a vegetarian way of life and needed a vegan diet low in calories to help them achieve their goals. The great news is that reducing one's intake of meat would result in low calorie consumption. The secret to making healthy vegan recipes is getting rid of the extra fat that makes meals substantial.

While making low-fat vegan dishes, folks should initially try to avoid using a lot of oil. For salads and tastings, one can still use extra virgin olive oil of the highest quality. EVOO provides some of the "beneficial fats" that our bodies require while having a lower calorie value.

In preparing vegetarian dishes with lower calorie counts, avoid eating fried items. Even if one does use the extra virgin olive oil for frying, one should avoid fried dishes as much as is practical because they typically contain more calories.

Steer clear of boiling the vegetables and instead steam them. Significant nutrients will be lost during boiling. For a change, grill some vegetables. To give them some moisture, you may also spritz on a low-calorie or light cooking spray, or even sprinkle some watery lemon juice on top.

If one must consume seafood due to their diet, boil the fish rather than frying it. It is recommended to grill the fish because it is a great way to add flavor and uniqueness to food. Spices are key components that can make a significant difference and offer a delicious and enticing low-fat vegetarian recipe.
Online resources abound for low-calorie vegetarian cooking. Cookbooks for vegetarians that contain low-fat recipes are also available. Simple substitutions like diet cheeses or plain yogurt for vinegary cream are a more efficient and practical way to create vegetarian recipes that are low in calories.

If a person is inventive, they will be astounded to learn that there are a ton of nutritious vegetarian meals available, and that they may incorporate these recipes into their diets to balance their weight loss goals.

All it takes is a little knowledge about substitutions that may be made to change high-calorie dishes into low-calorie foods with a little variation and lots of thought. Adopt low-calorie vegan dishes into your regular diet and realize that you may enjoy delectable cuisine while maintaining your vegetarian lifestyle.

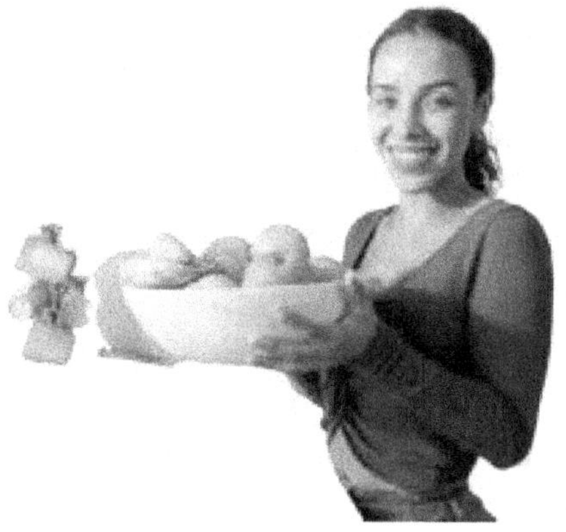

CHAPTER 7

Vegetarian Vegan

Since the dietary habits of vegetarians and non-vegetarians are unique and evident, the distinction between the two is well understood.

The distinction between vegetarianism and veganism is erroneously made, and there is another branch of the food-eating community that is popularly known as vegan. Although there are no obvious differences between vegan and vegetarian eating styles, many still struggle to classify these food eating groups.
You won't be able to distinguish between vegetarian and vegan diets as a layperson. Because of their evident and obvious similarities, people view these as belonging to the same food consumption groups.

People tend to believe what they see, therefore it's common to observe a vegetarian consuming fresh green salads and a few broccolini for each of their three meals. In actuality, not all vegetarians and vegans consume food in the same way and their practices are not necessarily complementary. Everything will become evident after you are aware of this faction's feeding habits. These are a few instances:

Lacto-ovo-vegetarians are people who eat dairy products, eggs, fruits, and vegetables. One of the most popular and common types of lacto-vegetarian diet is this one. These groups occasionally consume both fish and goods made from chicken.

Lacto-vegetarians consume dairy products, cereals, fruits, vegetables, and healthy nuts in their diet. The only distinction is that this group doesn't eat eggs.

Vegans: By observing their eating patterns, we can distinguish between vegans and vegetarians. Vegans refrain from consuming dairy products, eggs, or any other kind of animal products in their daily diet. These vegans have abstained from wearing or sporting anything made from animal products.

Macrobiotic: There are several benefits to sticking to a particular diet. Macrobiotic diet refers to a way of eating based on philosophy and spirituality. Before choosing this diet, health-related considerations are also taken into consideration. Foods are divided into negative and positive categories in this diet. Yang is the negative group, and ying is the positive group. This diet has many progression stages. At all levels, the use of animal products is promoted. The strictest level restricts consumption to only brown rice and bans even fruits and vegetables.

A typical person will undoubtedly mix up the vegetarian and lacto-vegetarian diets. But, adopting a vegan or vegetarian lifestyle is really simple. The benefits and drawbacks of a diet regimen become clear only once you begin to adhere to it. You should support any food eating regimens and diets as long as they are healthy and maintain you robust..